Carlos F. Quesada Molina
Ana Milena Muñoz
Marta Revelles Paniza

Fractures of the forearm, wrist, and hand

Carlos F. Quesada Molina
Ana Milena Muñoz
Marta Revelles Paniza

Fractures of the forearm, wrist, and hand

Diagnostic imaging and treatment

ScienciaScripts

Imprint
Any brand names and product names mentioned in this book are subject to trademark, brand or patent protection and are trademarks or registered trademarks of their respective holders. The use of brand names, product names, common names, trade names, product descriptions etc. even without a particular marking in this work is in no way to be construed to mean that such names may be regarded as unrestricted in respect of trademark and brand protection legislation and could thus be used by anyone.

Cover image: www.ingimage.com

This book is a translation from the original published under ISBN 978-620-3-03618-3.

Publisher:
Sciencia Scripts
is a trademark of
International Book Market Service Ltd., member of OmniScriptum Publishing Group
17 Meldrum Street, Beau Bassin 71504, Mauritius
Printed at: see last page
ISBN: 978-620-3-33266-7

INDEX

CHAPTER 1

ULNA AND RADIUS DIAPHYSEAL FRACTURES

DIAPHYSEAL FRACTURES OF BOTH BONES

Epidemiology

- Injury mechanism:
  - Direct: "*nightstick fracture*", by cane.
  - Indirect: fall with the arm in extension.
- Stress fractures in adults due to having suffered a fracture during childhood.
- Prolonged treatment with bisphosphonates.

Ranking

- AO:

- 2.2-A: simple fractures.
  - A1: radius intact.
  - A2: ulna intact.
  - A3: both bones affected.
- 2.2-B: fractures with third fragment.
  - B1: radius intact.
  - B2: ulna intact.
  - B3: one with third fragment, the other similar or simple.
- 2.2-C: complex fractures.
  - C1: complex ulna, simple radius.
  - C2: complex radius, simple ulna.
  - C3: both complex bones.

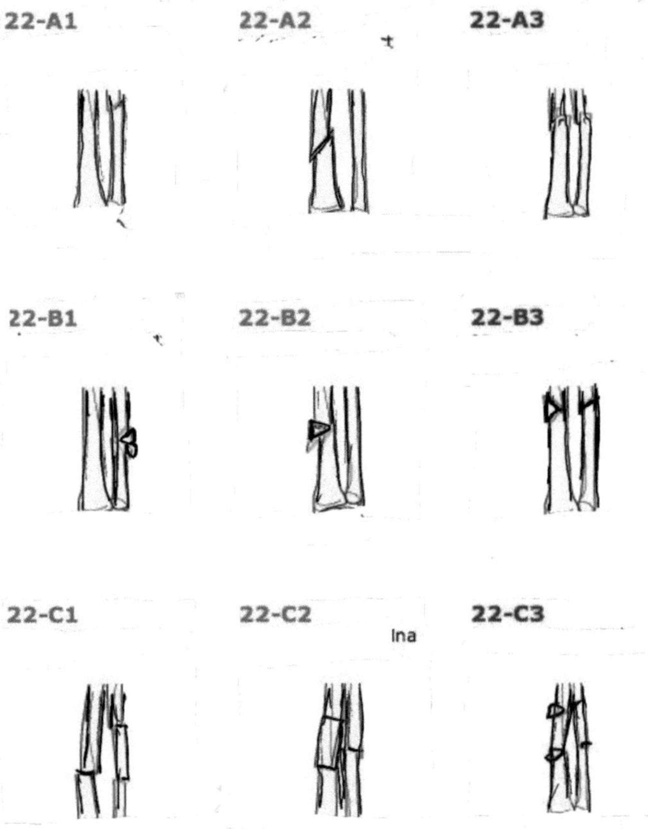

Image 1.1. AO classification.

Diagnosis

- Simple Rx:
    - Include distal and proximal radioulnar joint, to identify associated lesions.
    - These methods are used to diagnose rotational alterations after bone reduction:
        - Projection of the Evans bicipital tuberosity (medial if supination, posterior if neutral position and lateral if pronation).
        - Comparison of the thickness between the different radial fragments.
        - Opposite direction between the bicipital tuberosity and the radial styloid (AP projection in maximum supination).

- Crossed radius sign (crossing of both bones in an AP projection without maximum pronation).

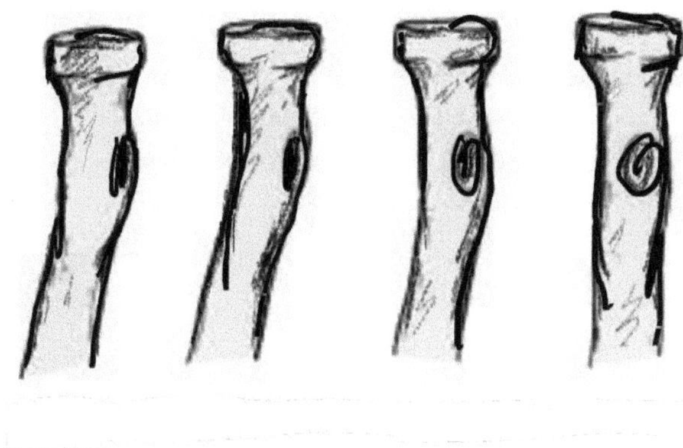

Position of the bicipital tuberosity.

- CT: to diagnose pseudarthrosis, rotational alterations and ARCD disruptions.
- MRI: to diagnose lesions of the ARCD.

Treatment

- The principles of articular fractures are applied:
  - Anatomical reduction.
  - Early mobilization.
- Alterations in the reduction may have repercussions on the range of motion of pronation.

- Non-displaced fractures:
  - Brachiopalmar cast in neutral pronation.
  - Change the plaster weekly.
  - Consolidation in 8-12 weeks.
- Displaced fractures:

- Best within the first 24 hours.
- Open reduction and osteosynthesis with interfragmentary compression plate (absolute stability).
- Include 6 cortices in each main fragment (3 screws).
- It is possible to use DCP (dynamic hole), LC-DCP (low contact) and LCP (screws locked to the plate) plates.
    - LCP plates have not demonstrated biomechanical or clinical superiority over DCP plates; they are useful in cases of severe osteoporosis.

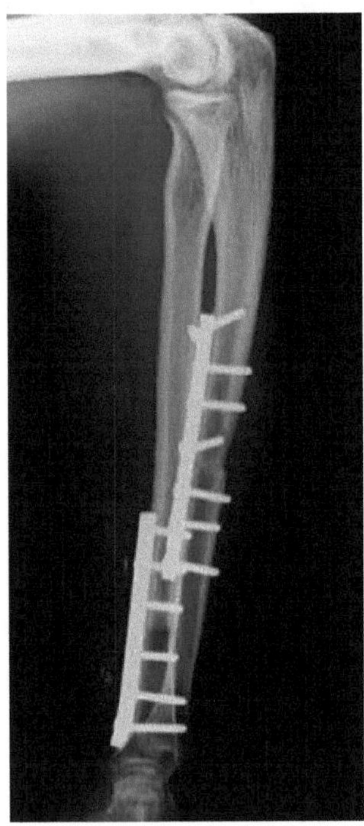

Image 1.3. X-ray showing an osteosynthesis with radius and ulna plates.

- It is preferable to perform a double incision to approach the radius and ulna, thus decreasing the risk of radioulnar synostosis.
- We should start with the bone that presents the least comminuted fracture, so that it will help us in the reduction of the other bone.
    - If both have complex fractures, start with the radius, which is the most complicated to reduce and in which both radial curves (supinator and pronator) must be restored.
    - Subcutaneous approach to the ulna.
    - Henry's volar approach for the radius (between the long supinator and palmaris major, from the radial styloid to the epicondyle) and Thompson's dorsal approach (for proximal radius fractures (from Lister's tubercle to the epicondyle).
    - To reduce the risk of compartment syndrome, the muscle fascia should not be closed.

- Early removal of the plaster splint and early mobilization.
- Removal of the osteosynthesis material after one year if there is discomfort and immobilization with a forearm orthosis to reduce the risk of refracture.
- Consolidation in 14 weeks.
- Intramedullary nails:
    - They do not achieve absolute stability, do not provide compression, and are used when:
        - Osteosynthesis with plates is not possible.
        - Children.
        - Prevention of pathological fractures.
    - Rotational disruptions are frequent.
    - Risk of injury to the posterior interosseous nerve (distal radius block in preformed nails).
    - Do not use Kirschner wires or Steinmann pins, due to loss of the pronator curve of the radius.
    - Consolidation 10 weeks (shorter than with plates).
    - Brachiopalmar plaster splint required.
- Hybrid fixation: radius plate and ulnar nail.

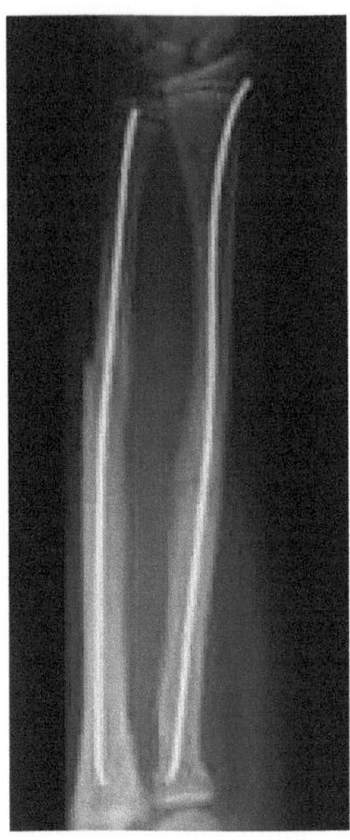

Nail system for infant diaphyseal radius and ulna fractures.

Complications

- Vicious consolidation: limiting pronosupination.
- Pseudarthrosis (up to 6% of fractures treated with plate).
- Predictable limitation of pronation (7° pronation, 9° supination) and loss of strength (up to 35%).
- Radio-ulnar synostosis: leads to a loss of pronation; especially if a single approach, elbow fractures or delayed surgery is performed.
- Compartment syndrome: the risk is increased if the muscle fascia is closed after osteosynthesis.
- Refracture: especially if there is early implant removal or if there has not been complete consolidation.
- Vascular lesions: if more than one vessel is affected, there is a risk of amputation; if one vessel is injured, the viability of the other arterial trunk must be checked.

ULNA DIAPHYSEAL FRACTURES

- They mainly affect young people due to direct trauma.
- More frequent in the middle and distal third.
- Fracture with displacement <50% or angulation <10°:
    - Brachiopalmar cast for 2 weeks, and brace for 12 weeks.
- Fracture with displacement >50% or angulation >10°:
    - Open reduction and internal fixation with plate.

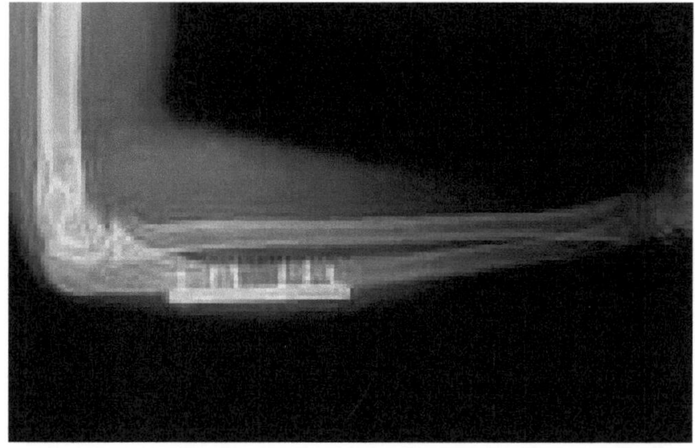

Image 1.5. Ulnar osteosynthesis with plate.

MONTEGGIA FRACTURE-LUXATION

- Ulna fracture + radial head dislocation.

Epidemiology

- Rare.
- Very underdiagnosed.

Ranking

➢ Bado:

- Type I: ulna fracture with anterior angulation + anterior dislocation of the radial head.
- Type II: ulna fracture with posterior angulation + posterior dislocation of the radial head.
- Type III: comminuted elbow fracture + lateral dislocation of the radial head.
- Type IV: ulna fracture + radius fracture + radial head dislocation.

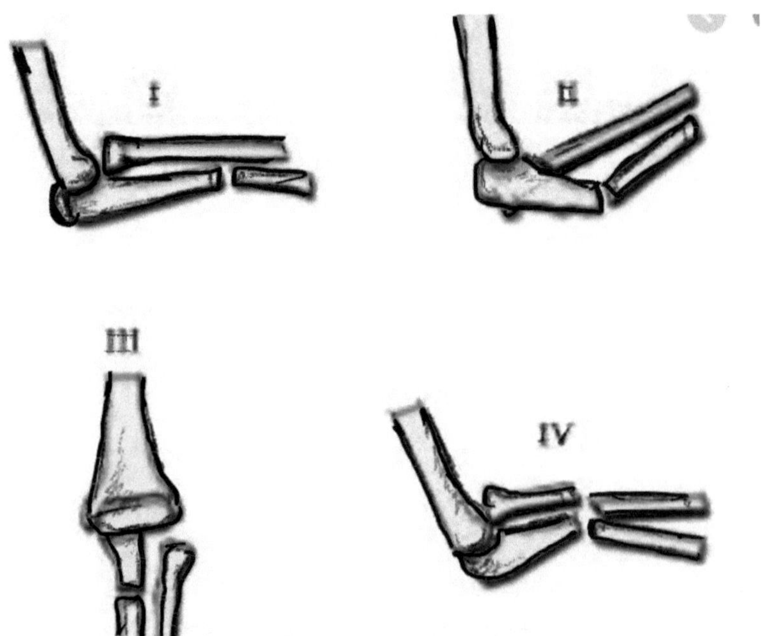

Figure 1.6. Bado's classification.

- Monteggia equivalents:

- Type I:
  - Anterior dislocation of the radial head.
  - Ulna fracture + radial neck fracture.
  - Radial neck fracture with anterior displacement.
  - Ulna fracture + more proximal radius fracture.
  - Ulna fracture + anterior radial head dislocation + olecranon fracture.
- Type II:
  - Dislocation of the radial head + fracture of the radial head epiphysis.
  - Radial neck fracture with posterior displacement.
- Type III (children):
  - Ulnar fracture in varus + fracture of the condyle.
- Type IV (children):
  - Distal humerus fracture + ulna fracture + radial neck fracture.

Clinic

- Ulna fracture + hemarthrosis (suspected).

Diagnosis

- Radial head dislocation: radiocapitellar alignment (the axis of the radius always points to the humeral condyle in all projections).

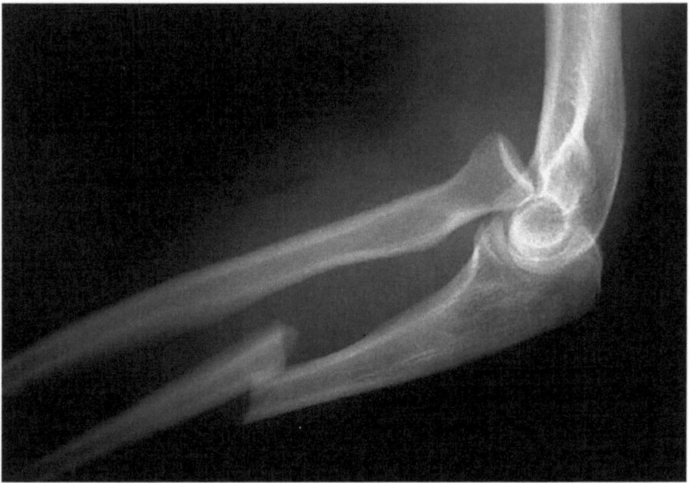

Image 1.7. Monteggia type I fracture-luxation.

Treatment

- Open reduction of the ulna and osteosynthesis with plate + closed reduction of the radial head.
    - If not reduced, open reduction with extension of Boyd's ulnar approach or independent approach (annular ligament, anterior capsule, anconeus).

      If not reduced, assess ulnar reduction.
- In cases of chronic dislocation of the radial head:
    - Open reduction and reconstruction of the annular ligament.
        - If not reduced, ulnar lengthening osteotomy.
            - If not reduced, radius shortening osteotomy.
    - Radial head excision.
- After reduction of the radial head:
    - If stable: plaster splint for 10 days.
    - If unstable: plaster splint until consolidation.

Complications

- High frequency.
- Posterior interosseous nerve injury: resolves spontaneously.

GALEAZZI FRACTURE-DISLOCATION

- Distal radius fracture + dislocation of the ARCD.

Epidemiology

- Very frequent.
- Middle-aged men.
- Instability:
    - Distal radius fracture.
    - Fracture of the base of the ulnar styloid.
    - Widening of the joint (AP).
    - Incongruence of the distal ulna (lateral).
    - Positive ulnar variance more than 5 mm.

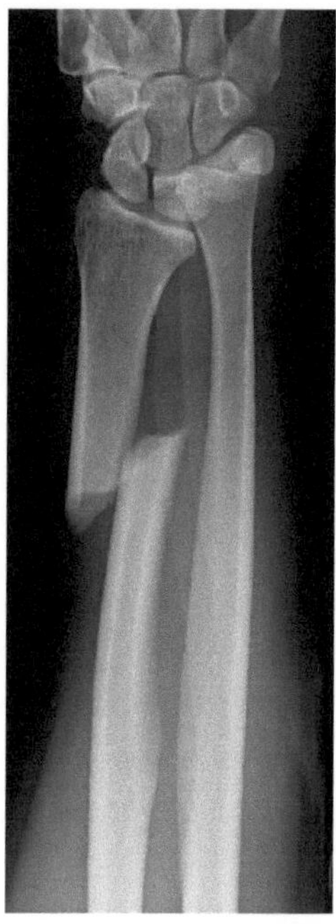

Image 1.8. Fracture-luxation of Galeazzi.

Treatment

- Open reduction of radius fracture + closed dislocation of ARCD.
- If not reduced, open reduction (triangular fibrocartilage).
- After reduction of ARCD:
    - If stable: brachiopalmar cast in medium pronosupination for 6 weeks.
        - If unstable: two radiocubital K-wires 6 weeks.

Complications

- Distal radioulnar pain.
    - Ulnar shortening if there is excessive positive ulnar variance.
    - ARCD fusion + proximal pseudoarthrosis.

CHAPTER 2

DISTAL RADIUS AND ULNA FRACTURES

Epidemiology

- They constitute 1/6 of all fractures of the body in adults.
- Peak incidence:
  - 5-15 years.
  - Males under 40 years old / Females over 40 years old.
- Production mechanism:
  - High-energy trauma: intra-articular fractures in men under 40 years of age.
  - Low-energy trauma: extra-articular fractures in women over 40 years of age.
  - They are usually falls with the support of the hand in extension; but they can also originate with the support of the hand in flexion, by axial compression or by shearing.

Diagnosis

- Main measurements on CXR to assess fracture displacement:
  - Radial length: 11mm.
  - Sagittal inclination: 11°.
  - Radial inclination: 21°.
- Additional screenings:
  - Lateral with ulnar tilt.
  - Tangential dorsl.
  - Oblique.

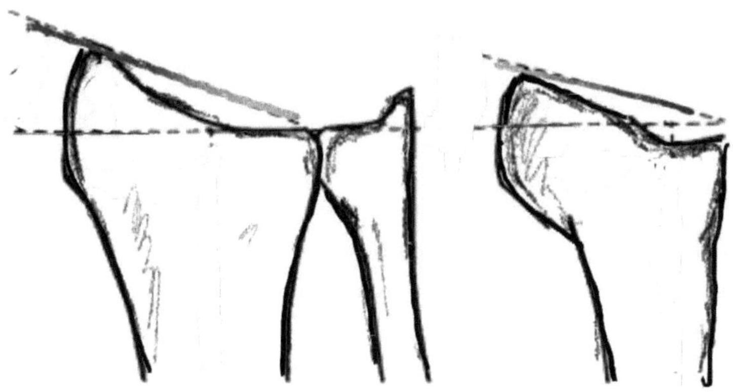

Image 2.1. Radiographic measurements of the displacement.

Ranking

➢ Classic eponyms:

- Colles: extra-articular with dorsal displacement.
- Smith: extraarticular with volar displacement.
- Barton: fracture-dislocation, dorsal or volar.
- Hutchinson / Chauffeur: styloid process of the radius.
- Die-Punch: lunate impaction.

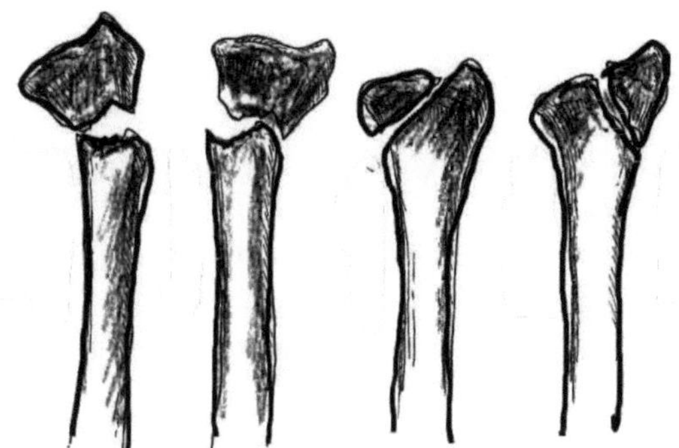

Image 2.2. Classical classification.

➢ Fernandez:

- I: metaphyseal fracture by flexion.
- II: joint fracture by shearing
- III: articular compression fracture.
- IV: avulsion fracture or fracture-dislocation fracture.
- V: high energy combined fracture.

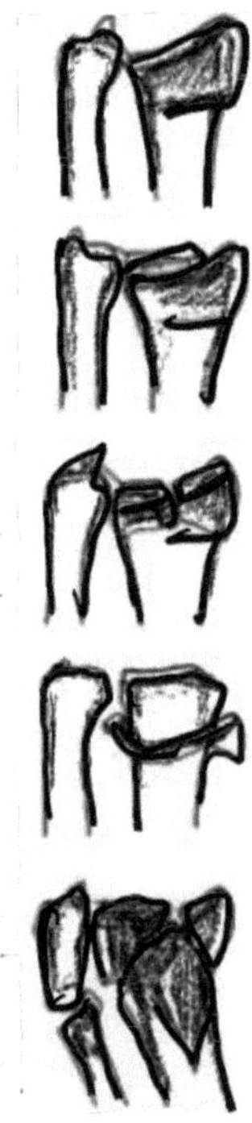

Image 2.3. Fernandez classification.

➢ Frykman:

- I: extra-articular distal radius fracture.
- II: extra-articular distal radius fracture + distal ulna fracture.
- III: fracture of the distal radius intra-articular radiocarpal distal radius.
- IV: intra-articular radiocarpal distal radius fracture + distal ulna fracture.
- V: fracture of the distal radius intra-articular radioulnar.
- VI: intra-articular distal radius fracture + distal ulna fracture.
- VII: intra-articular radicarpal and radioulnar distal radius fracture.
- VIII: intra-articular radiocarpal and radio-ulnar distal radius fracture + distal ulna fracture.

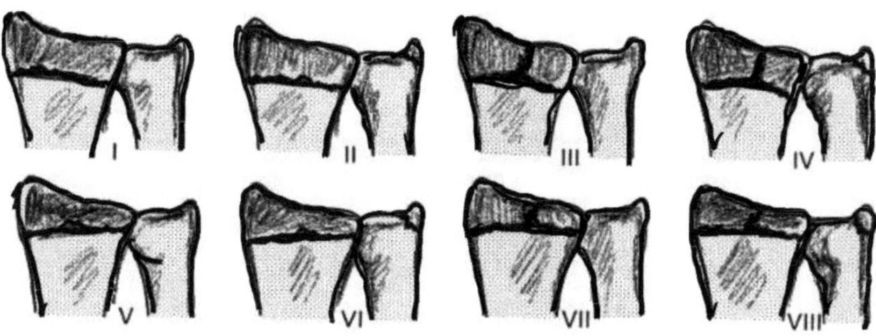

Figure 2.4. Frykman classification.

Instability criteria

- Age.
- Dorsal comminution or fracture of the distal ulna.
- Initial displacement:
    - > 10mm radial shortening.
    - > 20° of dorsal angulation.
- Secondary displacement.
- Intra-articular fracture.

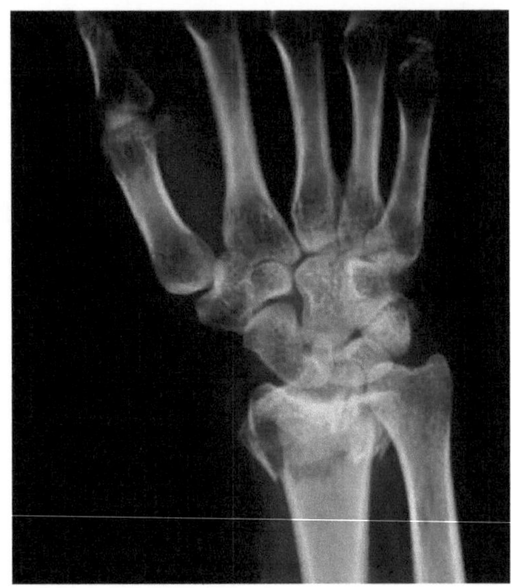

Image 2.5. Unstable radius fracture.

Associated injuries

- Scapholunate ligament: especially Hutchinson's fractures.
- Triangular fibrocartilage: suspect if there is radial shortening or dorsal angulation.
  - In such a case, place brachiopalmar cast in neutral position for 3 weeks.
- Distal radioulnar dislocation or instability.
- Median nerve: to prevent it, early reduction.
  - If not resolved within 48h, perform carpal tunnel decompression.
- Rupture of the extensor pollicis longus.

Treatment

- Closed plaster:
  - Indications:
    - Patients over 65 years of age with low functional demand.
    - Non-displaced fractures.
  - Change at 2 weeks to avoid cast loosening and secondary displacement.
  - Perform a weekly control X-ray within the first 3 weeks.

- Limits of closed reduction:
  - < 11° of dorsal angulation.
  - < 5mm radial shortening.
  - < 10° of radial inclination.
  - < 2mm of articular step.
- Maintain the cast for 6 weeks; in non-displaced patients, the immobilization period can be shortened to 4 weeks to reduce the risk of sympathetic algodystrophy and stiffness.

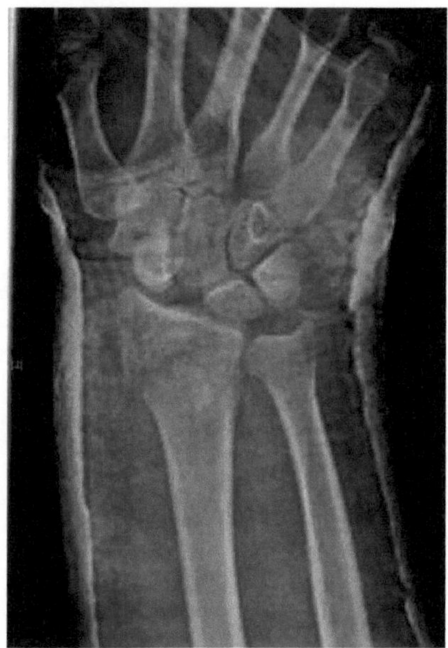

Image 2.6. Closed plaster.

- Kirschner needles:
  - Immobilization with plaster is always added.
  - Duration: 4 weeks.
  - Risk of injury to the sensory branch of the radial nerve and tendon injury.
  - Clancey:
    - A needle from radial styloid to dorsal.
    - A needle from radioulnar to volar.
  - Kapandji: 2 dorsal intrafocal needles and 1 or 2 radial intrafocal needles.

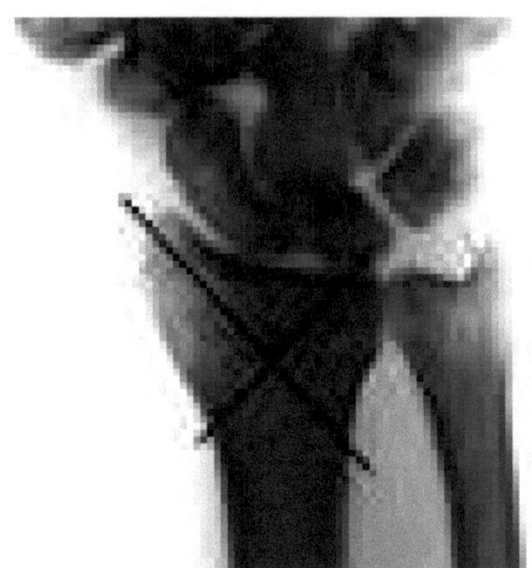

Image 2.7. Clancey.

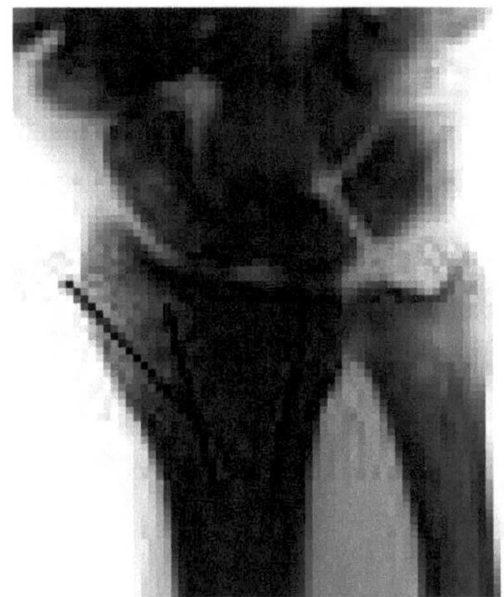

Image 2.8. Kapandji.

- Bipolar cast:
  - It consists of placing a needle in the second MTT and another in the radius, adding a plaster to maintain this length.
  - Disadvantages:
    - Pin infection.
    - Joint traction.
    - Indirect reduction.

        - No possibility of readjustment.

- External fixator:
    - o Between second MTT and radius or between radial diaphysis and distal fragment.
    - Indicated in extensive soft tissue lesions.
    - Avoid overdistraction to reduce the risk of stiffness.
- Flying plate:
    - Tenotomy of the supinator longus can be associated to facilitate fracture reduction, and the extended Orbay approach, freeing the first extensor compartment of the carpus.
    - o Plates of anatomical design, fixed or variable angle and screws locked to the plate are the most commonly used.
    - It is very important to reduce the ulnar part of the radius to minimize the risk of distal radioulnar instability.

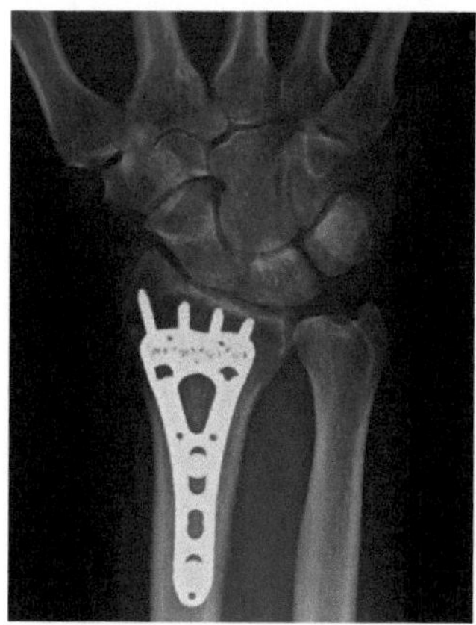

Image 2.9. Flying plate.

Complications

- Radiocarpal arthrosis: if there is a joint step > 2mm in young patients.
- Carpal tunnel syndrome.
- Sympathetic algodystrophy: due to a long period of immobilization.
- Secondary displacement and vicious consolidation: can lead to osteoarthritis.
    - Osteotomy is indicated as sequelae surgery if:
        - Radial shortening > 5mm.
        - Dorsal angulation > 20°.
        - Radial inclination < 10°.

CHAPTER 3

CARPAL FRACTURES

SCAPHOID FRACTURES

Epidemiology

- It is the most frequent fracture of the carpus (70%), and the second most frequent fracture of the wrist after the distal radius fracture.
- Many associated injuries.
- Mechanism of injury:
    - Axial load with the wrist in hyperextension.

Instability criteria

- Displacement > 1mm or transscaphoid angle >35°.
- DISI instability.
- Perilunate dislocations.
- Proximal pole.

Ranking

- According to location:
    - Middle third (the most frequent).
    - Distal third.
    - Proximal third (high incidence of absence of consolidation).
- According to stroke:
    - Transverse (60%).
    - Horizontal oblique.
    - Vertical oblique.

- Herbert:

- Type A: acute stable.
  - A1: distal tubercle.
  - A2: incomplete middle third.
- Type B: acute unstable.
  - B1: distal oblique.
  - B2: complete middle third.
  - B3: proximal pole.
  - B4: transscaphoid fracture-dislocation.
- Type C: delayed consolidation.
- Type D: pseudarthrosis.
  - D1: fibrous junction.
  - D2: pseudoarticulation.

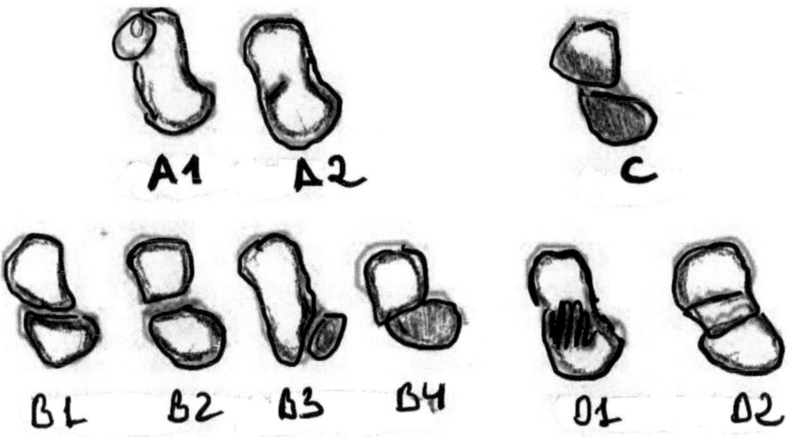

Image 3.1. Herbert's classification.

Clinic

- Patients with scaphoid fractures may be asymptomatic, although this is not the norm.
- Pain in the anatomical snuffbox, ulnar deviation and pronation.
- Painful axial compression of the first and second TCM.
- Hirsch's sign: painful axial compression of the third TCM with the wrist in radial deviation.

Diagnosis

- X-ray: If the radiographic tests are normal and the index of suspicion is high, the patient should be immobilized with a cast, and a control X-ray should be performed after a few weeks.
- MRI: early detection of scaphoid fracture in case the X-ray is negative. It is also useful for the assessment of osteonecrosis during follow-up.
- CT: to evaluate displacement and comminution.

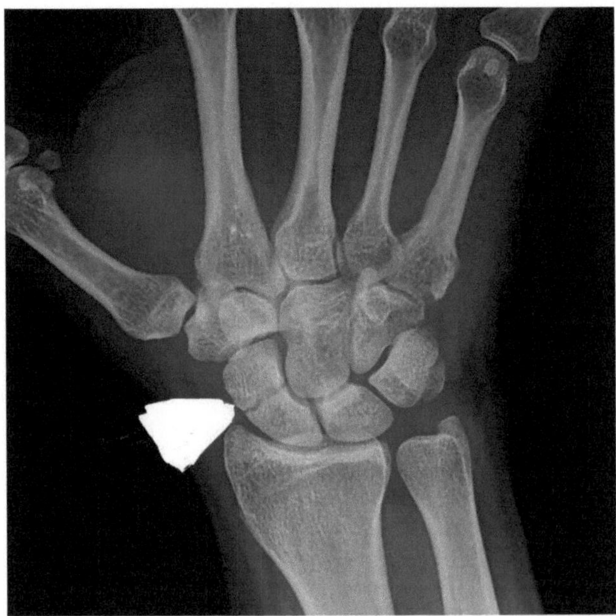

Image 3.2. Scaphoid fracture.

Treatment

- Non-displaced fractures:
  - Cast (including thumb) during:
    - Distal third: 2-3 months.
    - Middle third: 3-4 months.
    - Proximal third: 4-5 months.
- Unstable fractures:
  - Osteosynthesis with Herbert screw, mainly through a volar approach.

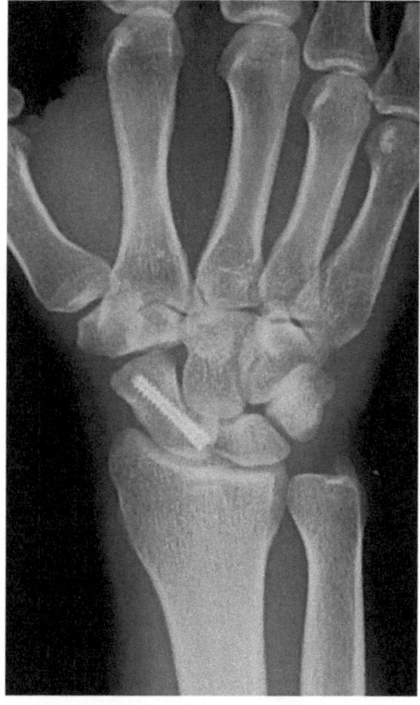

Image 3.3. Osteosynthesis of scaphoid fracture.

Complications

- Pseudarthrosis: occurs if there are no signs of healing more than 6 months after the fracture.
  - Most frequently, the middle third.
  - If the fracture is located distal to the dorsal-ulnar apex of the scaphoid, it is considered unstable, originating flexion of the distal fragment.

- Delay in treatment:
  - < 4 weeks: 5%.
  - > 4 weeks: 45%.
- Displaced fractures:
  - Surgical treatment: 1%.
  - Gypsum: 18%.
- Fractures of the proximal pole: 40%.
- CT and MRI.
- If asymptomatic, therapeutic abstention.
- Free bone graft with or without osteosynthesis / vascularized.

FRACTURES OF THE REST OF THE BONES

Fractures of the lunate

- After the scaphoid, they are the second most frequent fractures of the carpus.
- By fall with the support of the hand in hyperextension.
- Ulnar minus ulnar variance predisposes to lunate injury.
- MRI allows early detection of Kienböck's disease.
- Immobilization with plaster cast for 4 weeks.

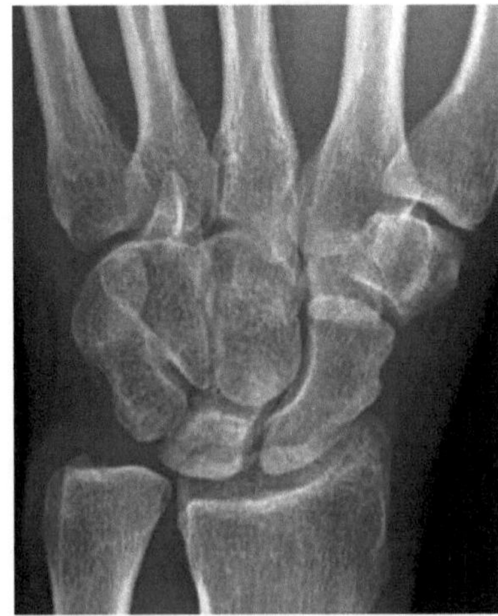

Image 3.4. Fracture of the lunate.

Hook fracture

- Direct trauma.
- The most frequent is the fracture of the hook of the hook, which is related to compression at the level of Guyon's canal.
- Ulnar artery and nerve injuries.
- Rx of the carpal tunnel.
- Osteosynthesis if the fragment is large, otherwise resect it.

Pyramidal fracture

- By impaction against the ulna.
- Falling with the wrist in ulnar deviation.

CHAPTER 4

HAND FRACTURES

FRACTURES OF THE DISTAL PHALANX

Epidemiology

- They make up 50%.
- The crushing of the distal phalanx stands out.

Treatment

- Crush fractures:
  - Conservative:
    - Immobilization with aluminum splint or cast.
    - Drainage of subungual hematoma.
    - Repair of the nail matrix.
- Displaced transverse fractures:
  - Surgical:
    - Closed reduction and needle fixation.
- Dorsal base fractures:
  - If there is involvement >25% of the articular surface or volar subluxation of the phalanx:
    - Closed reduction and needle fixation.
- Base volar fractures:
  - Surgical:
    - Open reduction and internal fixation (deep digital flexor avulsion).

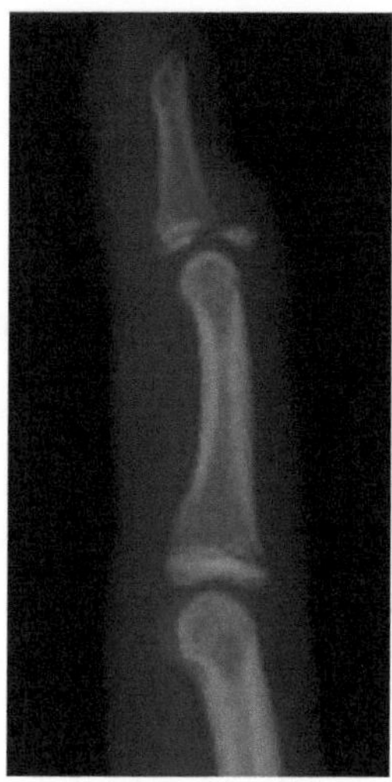

Image 4.1. Fracture of the distal phalanx.

DISTAL INTERPHALANGEAL DISLOCATIONS

- Pure dislocations:
    - Immobilization.
- Distal extensor tendon rupture:
    - Hyperextension immobilization with Stack splint (hammertoe prevention).
- Deep flexor tendon rupture:
    - Open reduction and osteosynthesis.

MIDDLE AND PROXIMAL PHALANX FRACTURES

- Fractures of the proximal phalanx tend to deform with volar angulation due to interosseous action.
- Proximal fractures of the middle phalanx angulate to volar while more distal fractures angulate to dorsal.

Treatment

- Non-displaced extra-articular fractures:
    - Syndactyly.
- Displaced extra-articular fractures:
    - Closed reduction and immobilization with syndactyly or intrinsic plus splint.

- Non-displaced intra-articular fractures:
    - Syndactyly.
- Displaced intra-articular fractures:
    - Angulation >10°, shortening >5mm.
    - Open reduction and internal fixation.
    - Dorsal approach for the proximal phalanx and medilateral approach for the middle phalanx.
    - If there is a lot of comminution at the base of the phalanx, traction can be applied using the Suzuki technique.
    - volar fractures of the base of the middle phalanx:
        - < 40% of the articular surface:
            - Splint immobilization with extension locking, starting from 60° flexion and increasing by 10° weekly.
    - Unicondylar fractures of the proximal phalanx:
        - Closed reduction and needle fixation.
        -

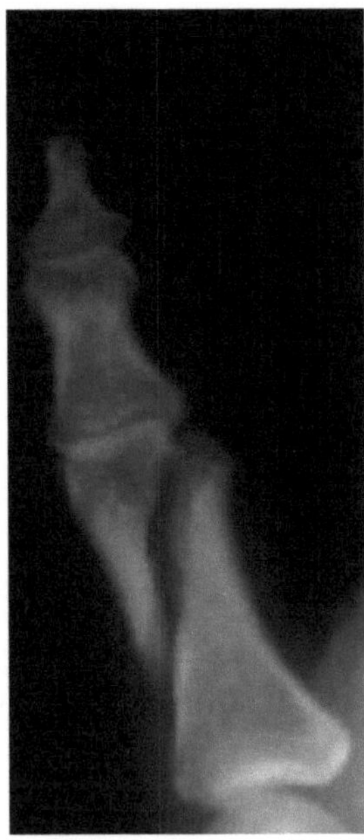

Image 4.2. Fracture of the proximal phalanx.

PROXIMAL INTERPHALANGEAL DISLOCATIONS

- Dorsal dislocation:
  - Constant volar plate breakage.
  - Syndactyly.
- Flying dislocation:
  - Central extensor tendon rupture.
  - Evolution to boutonnière deformity.
  - Boutonnière ferrule

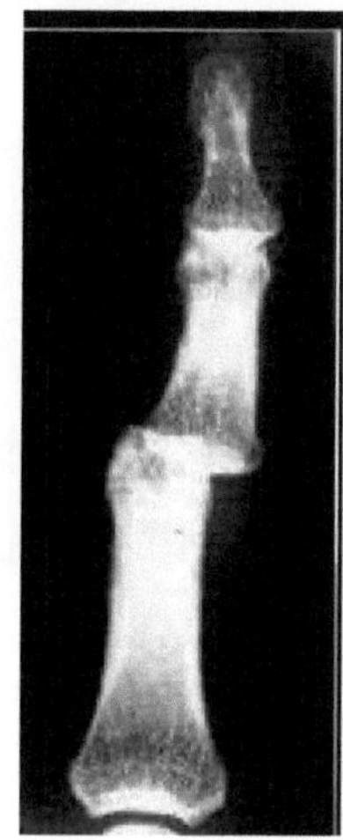

Image 4.3. Dislocation of the proximal interphalangeal joint.

METACARPOPHALANGEAL DISLOCATIONS

- Lateral dislocations:
  - Immobilization.
- Flying dislocations:
  - Surgical.
- Dorsal dislocations:
  - Closed reduction by hyperextension and posteriorly push distally.
  - If an attempt is made to reduce by longitudinal traction, the volar plate may be interposed, making it irreducible:
    - No obvious deformity.

- Flying skin retraction.
- Sesamoid in the joint space.
- Surgical treatment: volar approach.

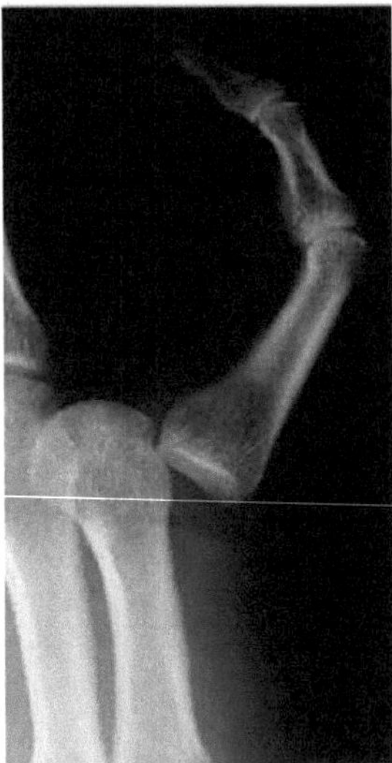

Image 4.4. Metacarpophalangeal dislocation.

METACARPAL FRACTURES

Fractures of the head

- Affection of the second MTC, especially.
- Intraarticular.
- Open reduction and internal fixation.

Neck fractures

- Affection of the fifth TCM, especially.
- If > 40° in the 4th and 5th MTC or > 10-15° in the 2nd and 3rd MTC:
    - Closed reduction using the Jahss technique: dorsal thrust with the finger flexed; and needles.

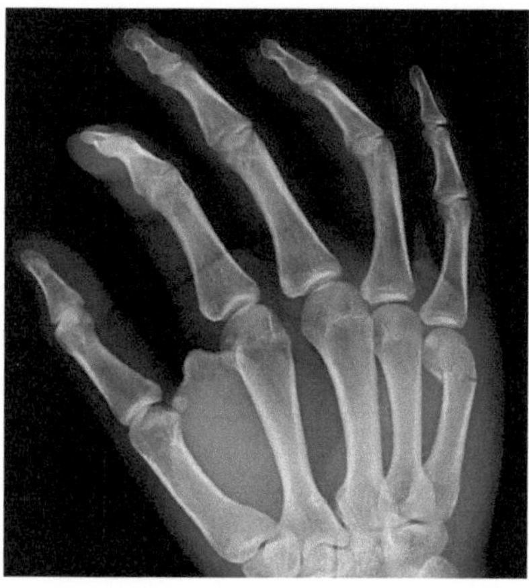

Figure 4.5 Metacarpal neck fracture.

Diaphysis fractures

- If > 20° in the 4th and 5th MTC or > 10° in the 2nd and 3rd MTC:
    - Closed reduction and needles.

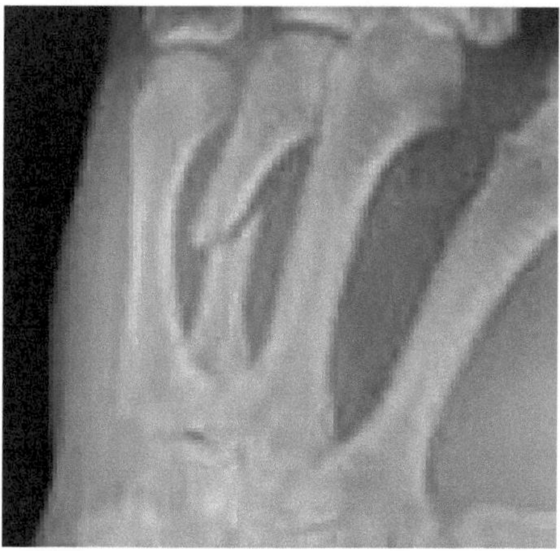

Image 4.6. Metacarpal diaphysis fracture.

Base fractures

- Stable, except 5th MTC:
    - Closed reduction and needles.
- Avulsion of the first and second radial at the base of the 2nd and 3rd MTC.

CARPOMETACARPAL DISLOCATIONS

- The most stable axis is the third TCM along with the large bone.
- Suspect metacarpal dislocation in the presence of a fracture with severe shortening of the adjacent TCM.
- It can be associated with carpal fracture.
- Dislocation of a TCM:
    - Closed reduction and needles.
- Dislocation of more than 2 MTC:
    - Open reduction and needles.

FRACTURES OF THE FIRST METACARPAL

- Extra-articular fractures:
    - These are the most frequent.
    - Conservative treatment.
    - If > 30° of angulation:
        - Closed reduction and plaster.

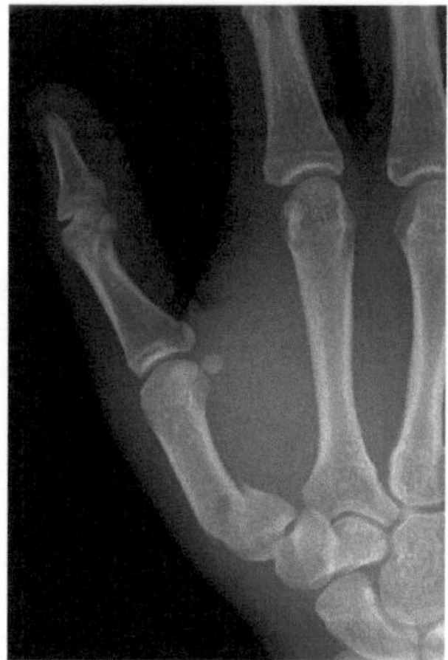

Image 4.7. Extra-articular fracture of the first MTC.

- Bennett's fracture:
  - It is an intra-articular fracture of simple trace.
  - Axial load with thumb in flexion
  - The thumb is shortened and adducted.
  - Closed reduction and pin fixation: traction with abduction, extension and pronation.

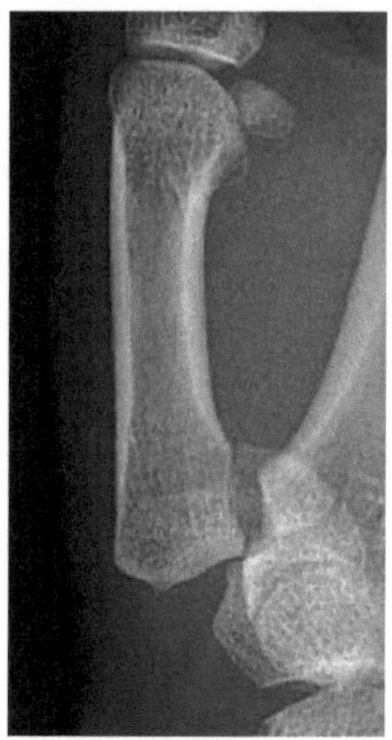

Image 4.8. Bennett's fracture.

- Rolando's fracture:
  - It is a complex intra-articular fracture.
  - T or Y fracture trace. Comminution.
  - Open reduction and internal fixation.

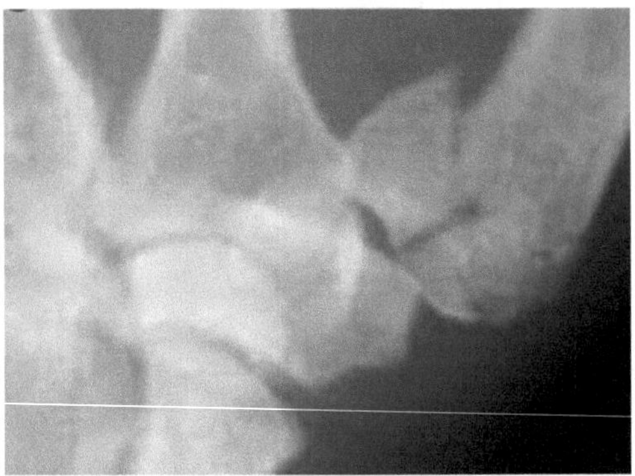

Image 4.9. Rolando's fracture.

METACARPOPHALANGEAL DISLOCATIONS

- Dorsal dislocation:
  - It is the most frequent.
  - Closed reduction.
  - If the plate is interposed fly:
    - Less conspicuous deformity.
    - Dimple in the skin.
    - Sesamoid in the joint.
    - Open reduction.
- Flying dislocation:
  - Surgical.

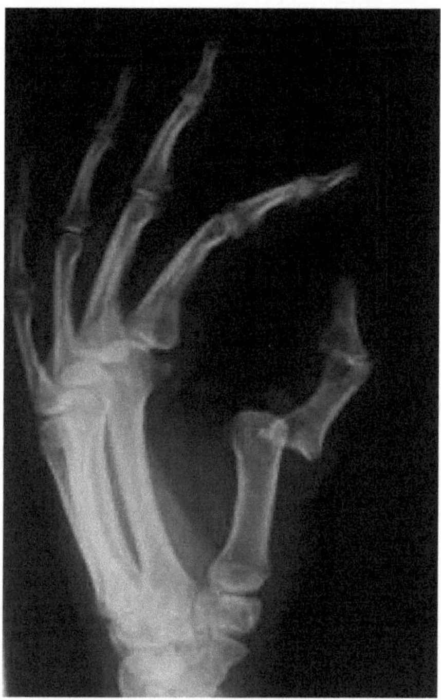

Figure 4.10. Metacarpophalangeal dislocation of the thumb.

Stener's lesion

- Also called "skier's finger" or "ranger's thumb".
- It is a lesion of the ulnar collateral ligament of the thumb.
- Produced by an abrupt abduction.
- Stener's lesion occurs when the adductor pollicis aponeurosis of the thumb is interposed.
- > 30° of forced valgus in flexion and extension or > 15° of valgus with respect to the contralateral.
- Partial ruptures:
    - Immobilization.
- Complete ruptures (instability in flexion and extension):
    - Surgical.

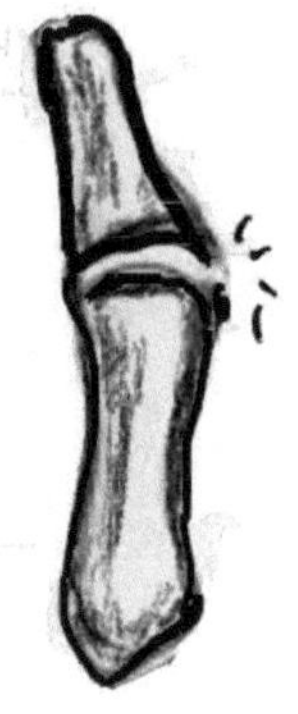

Image 4.11. Stener's lesion.

CARPOMETACARPAL DISLOCATIONS OF THE THUMB

- Infrequent.
- Poor prognosis.
- Dorsoradial and supination dislocation.
- Reduction with hyperpronation and fixation with needles.
- Chronic degenerative dislocations.

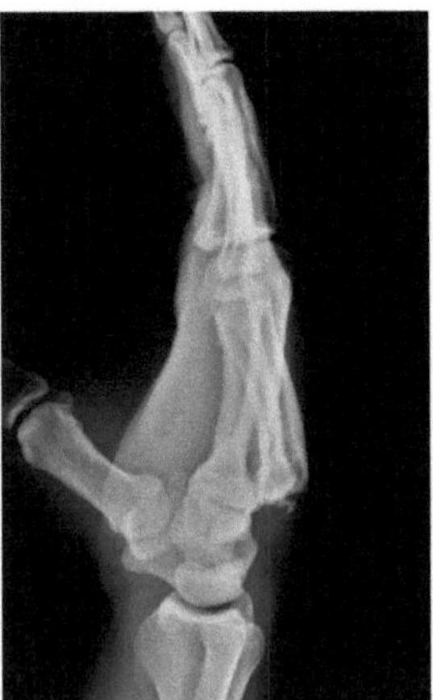

Figure 4.12. Carpometacarpal dislocation of the thumb.

BIBLIOGRAPHY

- Delgado Martínez AD. Orthopedic surgery and traumatology. 4th ed. Spain: Panamericana; 2018.
- Schünke M, Schulte E, Schumacher U, Voll M, Wesker K. Prometheus text and atlas of anatomy. Vol 2. 1st ed. Spain: Panamericana; 2005.
- Weiss DA. Master fractures in orthopedic surgery. 2nd ed. Spain: Marbán; 2009.
- McGinty JB, Burkhart SS, Jackson RW, Johnson DH, Richmond JC. Surgical arthroscopy. 3rd ed. Spain: Marbán; 2005.

-

-

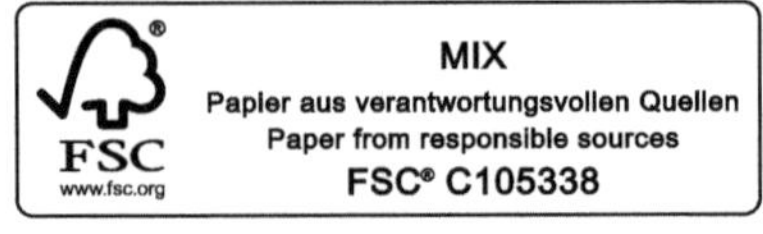

Printed by Books on Demand GmbH, Norderstedt / Germany